Blood sugar diet solution

The Comprehensive Guide to Stabilizing Blood Sugar and Improving Health"

LAUREN M. GREEN

TABLE OF CONTENT

INTRODUCTION

Chapter One

Chapter Two

Chapter Three

Chapter Four

Chapter Five

Chapter Six

Chapter Seven

Chapter Eight

Chapter Nine

Conclusion

INTRODUCTION

The Blood Sugar Diet is a revolutionary approach to managing diabetes and improving overall health. It is based on the latest scientific research and focuses on controlling blood sugar levels through a combination of healthy eating, regular exercise, and other lifestyle changes. By following this diet, individuals can reduce their risk of developing diabetes-related complications, improve their energy levels, and achieve a healthier weight. The Blood Sugar Diet is not a fad or a short-term solution, but rather a comprehensive plan for achieving long-term health and wellness.

Diabetes is a chronic condition characterized by high levels of sugar (glucose) in the blood. The two main types of diabetes are type 1 and type 2. In type 1 diabetes, the body does not produce enough insulin, a hormone that regulates blood sugar. In type 2 diabetes, the body does not produce enough insulin or does not use insulin properly.

Proper blood sugar management is essential for people with diabetes. This includes monitoring blood sugar levels, taking medications as prescribed, eating a healthy diet, and exercising regularly. People with diabetes may also need to use insulin injections or an insulin pump to help control their blood sugar levels.

Monitoring blood sugar levels can be done using a glucometer and test strips, which measure the amount of glucose in a small sample of blood. Keeping blood sugar levels within a healthy range can help prevent complications such as heart disease, nerve damage, and kidney damage.

If you have diabetes or suspect you may have it, it is important to speak with your healthcare provider for proper diagnosis and management. Diabetes is a chronic condition characterized by high levels of sugar (glucose) in the blood. The two main types of diabetes are type 1 and type 2. In type 1 diabetes, the body does not produce enough insulin, a hormone that regulates blood sugar. In type 2 diabetes, the body does not produce enough insulin or does not use insulin properly.

Proper blood sugar management is essential for people with diabetes. This includes monitoring blood sugar levels, taking medications as prescribed, eating a healthy diet, and exercising regularly. People with diabetes may also need to use insulin injections or an insulin pump to help control their blood sugar levels.

Monitoring blood sugar levels can be done using a glucometer and test strips, which measure the amount of glucose in a small sample of blood. Keeping blood sugar levels within a healthy range can help prevent complications such as heart disease, nerve damage, and kidney damage.

If you have diabetes or suspect you may have it, it is important to speak with your healthcare provider for proper diagnosis and management.

This guide will provide you with all the information you need to understand how the diet works, and how to implement it in your own life.

Chapter One

Understanding Blood Sugar

Blood sugar, also known as blood glucose, is the amount of sugar (glucose) present in the blood. Glucose is a vital source of energy for the body's cells and is carried to them via the bloodstream. The body regulates blood sugar levels through the actions of insulin, a hormone produced by the pancreas. When blood sugar levels are too high, the pancreas produces insulin to lower them, and when blood sugar levels are too low, the pancreas produces less insulin. Imbalances in blood sugar can lead to conditions such as diabetes.

How the body blood sugar levels

The body maintains blood sugar levels through a delicate balance of hormones and enzymes. The primary hormones involved in regulating blood sugar levels are insulin and glucagon, which are produced by the pancreas.

When you eat, the carbohydrates in your food are broken down into glucose, which enters the bloodstream and increases blood sugar levels. In response, the pancreas releases insulin, which helps to move glucose from the bloodstream into the cells of the body where it can be used for energy. Insulin also helps to store glucose in the liver and muscle tissue as glycogen, which can be converted back into glucose as needed.

When blood sugar levels fall too low, the pancreas releases glucagon, which signals the liver to convert stored glycogen back into glucose, which is then released into the bloodstream to raise blood sugar levels.

Other hormones such as Cortisol, Growth hormone and Somatostatin are also involved in regulating blood sugar levels. Additionally, enzymes such as glucose transporters and hexokinase play important roles in the uptake and utilization of glucose by the cells.

Overall, the body's blood sugar levels are constantly monitored and regulated through a complex interplay of hormones and enzymes to maintain a healthy balance.

Effects of high blood sugar

High blood sugar, also known as hyperglycemia, can lead to a variety of health problems if left untreated. Some of the short-term effects of high blood sugar include increased thirst and urination, blurred vision, fatigue, and slow wound healing. Long-term effects can include nerve damage, kidney damage, heart disease, and an increased risk of stroke. High blood sugar can also increase the risk of developing type 2 diabetes. It is important to monitor blood sugar levels and take steps to control them if they are consistently high. This can include making lifestyle changes, such as eating a healthy diet and getting regular exercise, as well as taking medication if prescribed by a doctor.

Effects of low blood sugar

Low blood sugar, also known as hypoglycemia, occurs when the level of glucose (sugar) in the blood is too low. This can happen if a person with diabetes takes too much insulin or other glucose-lowering medication, skips a meal, or exercises more than usual without adjusting their medication or food intake. Symptoms of low blood sugar include shakiness, sweating, confusion, difficulty speaking, and loss of consciousness. If left untreated, low blood sugar can lead to seizures or coma. It is important for people with diabetes to monitor their blood sugar levels regularly and take action to raise them if they become too low.

Chapter Two

The Blood Sugar Diet

The Blood Sugar Diet, also known as the low-carbohydrate diet, is a dietary approach that focuses on reducing the intake of carbohydrates in order to improve blood sugar control. The theory behind this diet is that by lowering carbohydrate intake, the body is forced to use fat as its primary source of fuel, which can lead to improved blood sugar control and weight loss. Some of the potential benefits of the Blood Sugar Diet include lower blood sugar levels, improved insulin sensitivity, and weight loss. However, it is important to note that the Blood Sugar Diet should be used under the guidance of a healthcare professional, as it may not be suitable for everyone and could lead to nutrient deficiencies if not properly followed.

An overview of the low-carbohydrate diet

A low-carbohydrate diet is a diet that limits the intake of carbohydrates, such as those found in sugary foods, pasta, and bread. The idea behind the diet is that by reducing the amount of carbohydrates consumed, the body will enter a metabolic state called ketosis, in which it begins to burn stored fat for energy instead of carbohydrates. This can lead to weight loss and other health benefits. However, it is important to note that the long-term safety and effectiveness of low-carbohydrate diets have not been extensively studied, and they may not be appropriate for everyone. Additionally, it is important to ensure that adequate amounts of essential nutrients are still consumed, and that the diet is tailored to individual needs and preferences.

Benefits for blood sugar control

There are several benefits to controlling blood sugar levels, including:

- Reducing the risk of diabetes and its complications, such as heart disease, stroke, kidney damage, and nerve damage.
- Improving energy levels and concentration.
- Helping to maintain a healthy weight.
- Reducing the risk of developing certain types of cancer.
- Improving overall health and wellbeing.

There are many different ways to control blood sugar levels, including diet, exercise, and medication. A healthcare professional can help you develop a plan that is tailored to your specific needs.

Chapter Three

Meal Planning: Tips and guidelines for planning healthy, blood sugar-friendly meals

When planning healthy, blood sugar-friendly meals, it's important to focus on nutrient-dense foods that are low in added sugars and refined carbohydrates. Here are some tips and guidelines to help you plan your meals:

- Prioritize non-starchy vegetables: Include a variety of vegetables in your meals, such as leafy greens, broccoli, cauliflower, bell peppers, and tomatoes. These are low in carbohydrates and high in fiber, vitamins, and minerals.

- Incorporate lean protein: Choose lean protein sources such as chicken, fish, tofu, and legumes. These can help keep you feeling full and satisfied, and can also help regulate blood sugar levels.

- Include healthy fats: Healthy fats such as avocado, olive oil, nuts, and seeds can help regulate blood sugar levels and keep you feeling full and satisfied.

- Limit added sugars and refined carbohydrates: Avoid foods and drinks that are high in added sugars, such as soda, candy, and processed snack foods. Additionally, limit your intake of refined carbohydrates, such as white bread and pasta.

- Plan ahead: Take the time to plan your meals and snacks in advance. This can help ensure that you have healthy options on hand when you need them, and can also help you avoid impulse eating.

- Consider using a meal delivery service: Many meal delivery services offer healthy and blood sugar-friendly options.

- Consult a dietitian or nutritionist: A dietitian or nutritionist can provide personalized recommendations for meal planning based on your individual needs and goals.

Chapter Four

Grocery Shopping and Meal Preparation

How to choose the right foods that support blood sugar control

Grocery shopping and meal preparation can play a big role in helping to control blood sugar levels. Here are a few tips to help you make healthy choices when shopping and preparing meals:

- Make a list: Plan out your meals and snacks for the week, and make a grocery list of the ingredients you will need. This will help you stay on track and avoid impulse purchases of high-sugar or high-carb foods.

- Shop the perimeter: The outer aisles of the grocery store typically have the freshest and most nutritious foods, such as fruits, vegetables, lean proteins, and whole grains. Try to limit your time in the inner aisles, where processed foods and snacks are often located.

- Read labels: Pay attention to the nutrition facts and ingredient lists of the foods you buy. Look for foods that are high in fiber, protein, and healthy fats and low in added sugars and refined carbohydrates.

- Cook at home: Preparing your own meals allows you to control the ingredients and portion sizes, which can be helpful for blood sugar control.

- Batch cook: Prepare larger portions of healthy meals and snacks, and store them in the refrigerator or freezer for later. This can save you time and make it easier to stick to your healthy eating plan when you're short on time.

- Consider the glycemic index (GI) of foods: when making food choices, choose foods with low-glycemic index, they will be absorbed slowly, helping to keep blood sugar levels more stable.

It's also important to consult with a healthcare professional to create an individualized plan that takes into account any health conditions, medications, and personal preferences.

How to prepare meals that support blood sugar control

To prepare meals that support blood sugar control, it's important to focus on nutrient-dense foods that are low in added sugars and refined carbohydrates. This includes:

- Eating plenty of non-starchy vegetables, such as leafy greens, broccoli, and cauliflower
- Incorporating healthy fats, such as olive oil, avocado, and nuts
- Choosing lean protein sources, such as chicken, fish, and legumes
- Incorporating whole grains, such as quinoa, brown rice, and whole wheat
- Limiting or avoiding processed foods, sugary drinks and snacks

- Eating meals at regular intervals and not skipping meals
- Eating slowly and listening to your body's signals of hunger and fullness

Additionally, it's important to work with a healthcare professional to determine your individual needs and any specific dietary restrictions you may have.

Chapter Five

Recipes: A collection of delicious, blood sugar-friendly recipes for breakfast, lunch, dinner, and snacks

A collection of delicious, blood sugar-friendly recipes typically includes dishes that are low in added sugars and refined carbohydrates, and high in fiber and nutrient-dense ingredients. These types of recipes can help individuals with diabetes or blood sugar imbalances manage their condition by keeping blood sugar levels stable. Some examples of blood sugar-friendly foods include leafy greens, berries, nuts, and lean proteins like chicken and fish. Recipes in this collection might include meals such as roasted vegetable salads, grilled fish with a side of quinoa, or berry and almond smoothie bowls.

A collection of delicious, blood sugar-friendly recipes for breakfast.

A collection of delicious, blood sugar-friendly recipes for breakfast may include:

- Spinach and feta omelette: Whisk together eggs, spinach, and feta cheese, and cook in a skillet for a high-protein breakfast that's low in refined carbohydrates.

- Blueberry and almond smoothie: Blend together frozen blueberries, almond milk, almond butter, and a scoop of protein powder for a satisfying breakfast smoothie.

- Avocado toast with poached egg: Toast a slice of whole-grain bread and top with mashed avocado and a poached egg for a healthy and delicious breakfast.

- Greek yogurt parfait: Layer Greek yogurt, berries, and chopped nuts in a jar for a high-protein breakfast that's low in added sugars.

- Chia seed pudding: Mix together chia seeds, almond milk, vanilla extract, and a pinch of cinnamon and let sit overnight in the refrigerator for a healthy breakfast option.

- Breakfast burrito: Scramble eggs with veggies, like spinach, tomatoes, and bell peppers, and wrap in a whole wheat tortilla.

- Breakfast bowl: Cook up a batch of steel-cut oats, and top with your choice of fresh fruits, nuts and seeds, and a drizzle of maple syrup for a healthy and satisfying breakfast.

These recipes are just a few examples of the many delicious and blood sugar-friendly breakfast options that are available. It's important to consult with a healthcare professional to find the best options for you, depending on your specific health condition.

A collection of delicious, blood sugar-friendly recipes for lunch.

Here are three delicious, blood sugar-friendly recipes for lunch:

Grilled Chicken Salad:

- Grill 4 chicken breasts and slice them into strips.
- In a large bowl, toss together mixed greens, sliced cucumbers, cherry tomatoes, and sliced red onions.
- Add the chicken strips and toss to combine.
- For the dressing, mix together 2 tablespoons of olive oil, 1 tablespoon of apple cider vinegar, and a pinch of salt and pepper.
- Drizzle the dressing over the salad and enjoy.

Turkey Lettuce Wraps:

- In a pan, cook 1 pound of ground turkey with 1 diced onion, 2 cloves of minced garlic, and 1 diced red pepper.

- Once the turkey is cooked through, add in 2 tablespoons of soy sauce, 1 tablespoon of rice vinegar, and 1 teaspoon of sesame oil.
- Serve the turkey mixture in lettuce cups and top with chopped cilantro and green onions.

Black Bean Soup:

- In a pot, sauté 1 diced onion, 2 cloves of minced garlic, and 1 diced red pepper in a tablespoon of olive oil.

- Add 1 can of black beans, 1 cup of chicken or vegetable broth, 1 cup of diced tomatoes, 1 teaspoon of cumin, and 1 teaspoon of chili powder.

- Bring the mixture to a boil and then reduce the heat and let it simmer for 10 minutes.

- Serve the soup with a squeeze of lime juice, and a dollop of sour cream.of diced tomatoes, 1 teaspoon of cumin, and 1 teaspoon of chili powder.

- Bring the mixture to a boil and then reduce the heat and let it simmer for 10 minutes.

- Serve the soup with a squeeze of lime juice, and a dollop of sour cream.

A collection of delicious, blood sugar-friendly recipes for Dinner.

Here are a few blood sugar-friendly dinner recipe ideas:

- Grilled chicken with a side of roasted vegetables (such as broccoli, cauliflower, or green beans)

- Baked salmon with a side of quinoa or brown rice

- Turkey chili made with lean ground turkey, kidney beans, tomatoes, and spices (such as cumin and chili powder)

- Vegetable stir-fry made with your choice of vegetables (such as bell peppers, onions, and carrots) and a lean protein (such as chicken, shrimp, or tofu)

- Grilled pork tenderloin with a side of roasted sweet potatoes

- Black bean and vegetable enchiladas

- A salad with mixed greens, topped with grilled chicken or shrimp, avocado, and a vinaigrette dressing

- Spaghetti Squash with Turkey Meatballs

All of these recipes can be adjusted to your taste and dietary needs. You can also experiment with different herbs and spices to add flavor without adding sugar. Remember to also include a balanced amount of carbs, protein and healthy fats in your meals.

A collection of delicious, blood sugar-friendly recipes for snacks

Here are a few blood sugar-friendly snack recipe ideas:

- Greek yogurt with fresh berries and a drizzle of honey or a sprinkle of cinnamon

- Whole grain crackers with hummus or guacamole

- Apple slices with almond butter

- Cucumber and tomato slices with a sprinkle of feta cheese and a drizzle of balsamic vinegar

- Hard-boiled eggs

- Veggie sticks with a low-fat ranch dressing or salsa

- Edamame with a sprinkle of sea salt

- A smoothie made with Greek yogurt, frozen berries, and a scoop of protein powder

- Baked sweet potato chips

- A small serving of nuts (almonds, walnuts, pecans)

All of these recipes are high in fiber and protein, and low in added sugars, which can help keep blood sugar levels stable. You can also experiment with different herbs and spices to add flavor without adding sugar. Remember to also include a balanced amount of carbs, protein and healthy fats in your snacks.

Chapter Six

Lifestyle changes

How to make other lifestyle changes that can support blood sugar control.

In addition to eating a healthy diet, other lifestyle changes that can help support blood sugar control include:

Exercise: Regular physical activity can help lower your blood sugar levels and improve your overall health. Aim for at least 30 minutes of moderate-intensity exercise, such as brisk walking, cycling, or swimming, most days of the week. If you have been inactive for a while, start with shorter periods of exercise and gradually increase the duration and intensity.

Stress management: Stress can cause your blood sugar levels to spike, so it's important to find ways to manage stress. Techniques such as yoga, meditation, deep breathing exercises, or even taking a walk in nature can help reduce stress and improve your overall well-being.

Quitting smoking: Smoking increases your risk of developing diabetes and other health problems.

Sleep: Getting enough sleep is essential for maintaining blood sugar control. Aim for 7-9 hours of sleep each night and try to go to bed and wake up at the same time every day. Avoid caffeine and electronic devices before bed to help you relax and fall asleep faster.

Mindfulness: Incorporating mindfulness practices like meditation, yoga, or tai chi can help you to manage stress, improve sleep, and be more aware of your body, which can help you to make healthier food choices.

Social Support: Surround yourself with friends and family who encourage healthy behaviors, and seek out support groups or online communities of people with similar goals.

Time Management: Prioritize and plan out your day, to reduce stress and make time for exercise, sleep, and healthy meals.

It's important to note that everyone is different and what works for one person may not work for another. It's important to consult with a healthcare professional or a registered dietitian before making any drastic changes to your lifestyle.

Chapter Seven

Monitoring and Managing Blood Sugar

Monitoring and managing blood sugar, also known as blood glucose, is an important aspect of maintaining overall health and preventing complications related to diabetes. Blood sugar levels can be affected by a variety of factors, including diet, physical activity, medications, and stress.

Regularly monitoring blood sugar levels through a glucometer and keeping track of the results can help individuals with diabetes or those at risk of developing diabetes to understand how different factors affect their blood sugar levels. This information can then be used to make adjustments to diet, exercise, and medications to help maintain healthy blood sugar levels.

Managing blood sugar also involves making lifestyle changes to improve overall health and prevent the development of diabetes or complications related to diabetes. This includes eating a healthy diet, getting regular physical activity, managing stress, getting enough sleep, drinking alcohol in moderation, and maintaining a healthy weight.

It is important to consult with a healthcare professional or a registered dietitian to develop an individualized plan for monitoring and managing blood sugar. They can help to guide you on the best way to monitor and manage your blood sugar level.

How to use glucose meters to manage and monitor blood sugar

A glucose meter is a device used to measure the amount of glucose, or sugar, in the blood. It is a small, portable device that can be used at home or on the go to monitor blood sugar levels. Here are the steps for using a glucose meter:

- Obtain a small drop of blood from your fingertip using a lancet, a small device that pierces the skin to obtain a small drop of blood.

- Place the blood drop on a test strip, which is a small strip of paper or plastic that is inserted into the glucose meter.

- Follow the instructions on the glucose meter to insert the test strip and obtain a reading. The reading will typically appear on a digital screen within a few seconds.

- Record the reading and the time it was taken in a logbook or a mobile application.

- Compare the reading with the normal range for blood sugar levels, which is typically between 70-130 mg/dL before a meal and less than 180 mg/dL after a meal. If the reading is outside of this range, consult with a healthcare professional or a registered dietitian to understand why and adjust your treatment plan accordingly.

- Repeat the process as often as recommended by your healthcare provider, typically before and after meals and at bedtime.

It's important to note that each glucose meter may have different instructions and may require different test strips, so it's important to carefully read the instructions for your specific meter and follow them closely. Additionally, it is important to regularly calibrate your glucose meter to ensure accurate results.

How to track blood sugar levels

Tracking your blood sugar levels is an important part of managing and monitoring your diabetes or prediabetes. Here are some steps you can take to track your blood sugar levels:

- Use a glucose meter to measure your blood sugar levels at regular intervals, as recommended by your healthcare provider. This typically includes before and after meals, and at bedtime.

- Keep a logbook or use a mobile application to record your blood sugar readings, along with the time they were taken, the type of activity you were doing, and what you ate.

- Use the logbook or application to track patterns and trends in your blood sugar levels, such as how they are affected by different types of food, physical activity, and medications.

- Share your logbook or application data with your healthcare provider, so they can help you understand your blood sugar patterns and make adjustments to your treatment plan as needed.

- Take note of any symptoms you may have when blood sugar is high or low, such as sweating, weakness, confusion, or blurred vision.

- Review your logbook or application on a regular basis with your healthcare provider, and make any necessary adjustments to your treatment plan, such as medication dosages or meal plans.

- Keep a copy of your logbook or application data with you in case of emergencies, so medical personnel can quickly access your medical history.

It's important to note that everyone is different, and what works for one person may not work for another. It's important to consult with a healthcare professional or a registered dietitian to develop an individualized plan for monitoring and managing blood sugar.

How to adjust medication to support blood sugar level

There are several ways to adjust medication to support blood sugar levels, including:

- Changing the dose: Your healthcare provider may adjust the dose of your medication based on your blood sugar levels.

- Switching to a different medication: If your current medication is not working effectively, your healthcare provider may switch you to a different medication that may better control your blood sugar levels.

- Combining medications: Your healthcare provider may prescribe a combination of medications to help control your blood sugar levels.

- Monitoring blood sugar levels regularly: Your healthcare provider will likely ask you to check your blood sugar levels at home and bring a record of your levels to your appointments. This will help them determine if your medication needs to be adjusted.

It is important to remember that medication adjustments should only be made under the guidance of a healthcare provider and not self-adjusted.

Chapter Eight

Coping with challenges: How to manage common challenges that can arise when following a blood sugar diet.

Here are a few strategies for managing common challenges that can arise when following a blood sugar diet, such as eating out, dealing with cravings, and managing blood sugar during special occasions:

- Eating out: When eating out, look for options that are high in protein and fiber and low in added sugars and refined carbohydrates. Avoid deep-fried foods and opt for grilled or baked options instead.

- Dealing with cravings: Cravings for sugary or high-carb foods can be difficult to resist. To manage cravings, try keeping healthy snacks on hand, such as nuts, seeds, or fresh fruit, and engage in stress-relieving activities, such as exercise or meditation.

- Managing blood sugar during special occasions: Special occasions, such as holidays and parties, can be a challenge when following a blood sugar diet. To manage your blood sugar levels during these occasions, try to stick to your usual meal schedule as much as possible, eat a small, healthy snack before the event, and limit your intake of high-sugar or high-carb foods.

- Be prepared for unexpected situations: Pack a healthy snack with you, such as nuts or seeds, and keep a glucose meter with you to check your blood sugar levels as needed.

- Avoiding high-carb foods and added sugars: Foods such as white bread, white pasta, and sugary drinks can cause your blood sugar levels to spike. Try to limit your intake of these foods and opt for whole grains and natural sweeteners instead.

- Use a plate method: Use a plate method when eating, which is a visual guide to a healthy meal, filling half of the plate with non-starchy vegetables, a quarter with a protein-rich food, and a quarter with a whole grain or starchy vegetable.

- Make healthy substitutions: Instead of white flour, use almond flour, chickpea flour or cauliflower rice. Instead of sugar, use natural sweeteners like honey, maple syrup or stevia.

- Communicate with friends and family: Let your friends and family know about your dietary restrictions and ask for their support. They can help you make healthier choices and avoid temptations.

- Eat regularly and don't skip meals: Skipping meals can cause your blood sugar levels to drop too low, so make sure to eat regular meals and snacks throughout the day.

- Seek support from a registered dietitian or a diabetes educator: They can help you create a meal plan that meets your specific needs and can provide guidance for managing your blood sugar levels during special occasions.

Chapter Nine

Summary of the key takeaways and tips for success on a blood sugar diet.

A blood sugar diet, also known as a low-glycemic diet, is a dietary plan that focuses on limiting the intake of foods that cause a rapid spike in blood sugar levels. The key takeaways and tips for success on a blood sugar diet include:

- Choose low-glycemic foods: These include fruits, vegetables, whole grains, and lean proteins. These foods are digested more slowly and cause a slower rise in blood sugar levels.

- Avoid high-glycemic foods: These include processed foods, sugary drinks, and foods made with refined flour. These foods are digested quickly and cause a rapid spike in blood sugar levels.

- Eat regular, balanced meals: Eating regular, balanced meals throughout the day can help stabilize blood sugar levels and reduce cravings for high-glycemic foods.

- Incorporate healthy fats: Healthy fats such as olive oil, avocado, and nuts can slow the absorption of carbohydrates and help stabilize blood sugar levels.

- Be mindful of portion sizes: Consuming large portions of any type of food can cause a spike in blood sugar levels, so it's important to be mindful of portion sizes when following a blood sugar diet.

- Exercise regularly: Regular physical activity can help lower blood sugar levels and improve overall health.

- Consult with a healthcare professional: Before starting any new diet, it's always a good idea to consult with a healthcare professional to ensure that it's the right fit for you and your specific health needs.

Conclusion

In conclusion, a blood sugar diet is a dietary plan that focuses on limiting the intake of foods that cause a rapid spike in blood sugar levels. By choosing low-glycemic foods, avoiding high-glycemic foods, eating regular balanced meals, incorporating healthy fats, being mindful of portion sizes, exercising regularly and consulting with a healthcare professional, one can follow a blood sugar diet successfully. Following a blood sugar diet can help stabilize blood sugar levels, reduce cravings for high-glycemic foods and improve overall health. It is important to note that, as with any diet, individual results may vary and it's always a good idea to consult with a healthcare professional before making any significant changes to your diet or lifestyle.

www.ingramcontent.com/pod-product-compliance
Lightning Source LLC
Chambersburg PA
CBHW061606250726

48657CB00017B/2155